What to eat

for a long Life

Do you want to enjoy life?
Do you want renewed youth?
You want an attractive appearance
Do you want fitness

If so then live life properly Think about what you will
eat and what you will drink, but properly

What to eat

for a long Life

Do you want to enjoy life?
Do you want renewed youth?
You want an attractive appearance
Do you want fitness

If so then live life properly Think about what you will eat and what you will drink, but properly

d.ROJINA SALADIN

Presentation

When you seek to lose weight, to look as you like, you may find it difficult or no one will help you. This does not mean that you have to surrender. Maintaining proper weight is not only important to your well-being and personal satisfaction, it can be a reason for your constant happiness. It is not difficult, just the will.They need to eat nutrients in small amounts and more and more nutrients

However, we should realize that the urpose of weight gain, must be for logical reasons

If you're not successful before, we can let you get back on track and get well with these 14 steps to lose weight and keep it off.

There was a problem in the nature of life, individuals ate binge They go to work.

In the past society was better than the current society because the work was not behind the PC screen, but on their feet in the fields or factories

The most horrifying thing is that most of this weight gain is due to lifestyle, and the more dangerous it is moving towards becoming. Overweight increases the disease, regardless of diabetes or heart, it is binding

This eBook is your manual for losing that initial ten pounds that we as a whole battle with. It's astounding what little changes throughout your life can signify you shedding ten pounds and they all spin around eating right and getting your body moving .

Section 1

Weight reduction starting with what you drink

As a matter of first importance, individuals don't understand that what they drink is the initial phase in losing that initial 10 pounds. Truth be told, the vast majority don't have the foggiest idea about that when they feel hungry, they may really be dried out and they are extremely parched, not ravenous. Water is noteworthy also. Over 66% of your body weight is only water. This is additionally why water assumes an essential job in weight control. So TIP #1 is :

Drink a lot of water. It is suggested that you drink 8 glasses for each day, yet that may set aside you some opportunity to work up to. Your body needs a mess of water. Water doesn't simply flush every one of the poisons out of your body, however it improves you feel and more advantageous. When you drink a great deal of water you simply start to feel fit and this is the inspiration you have to get more fit .

The best thing about water is you can drink as much as you need since it has no calories by any means. When you're drinking a great deal of water, you eat less also in light of the fact that you won't feel just as you are starving to death. Keep in mind, on the off chance that you feel hungry, have a go at drinking a glass of water first and you'll understand you were most likely simply dried out and not ravenous by any means .

The entire 8 glasses multi day rule is truly something you ought to make progress toward. The most ideal approach to do this and to gauge your water admission is to purchase a container from the medication store or supermarket that is intended to hold precisely 8 glasses of water. These are incredible weight reduction devices since you can top them off, solidify them and as it dissolves for the duration of the day you have new and chilly water. Or then again, if its all the same to you your water room temperature you can drink it that path too. The only thing that is in any way important is that you're getting in the water your body needs .

TIP #2: Start off your day with a crisp, clean glass of water. When you get up in the first part of the day, drink one down. This will assist your body with getting going in light of the fact that it won't battle through lack of hydration. Likewise, after you drink a glass of water you won't have to have such a substantial breakfast. A glass of water awakens all the stomach related squeezes in your body and gets it all around greased up. You can generally have your morning espresso or tea, yet make certain to have a glass of water a short time later. Caffeine gets dried out you and you need to avoid lack of hydration .

TIP #3: Drink a glass of water before you take a seat to eat. Water will normally make you feel more full so you don't need to eat as much nourishment .

TIP #4: Have a glass of water while you eat also. Take a beverage after each nibble and you will feel full more rapidly so you can leave the table inclination fulfilled without feeling enlarged. Drinking water while you eat will likewise assist your nourishment with settling all the more rapidly, which additionally encourages you to feel full quicker .

TIP #5: Do your best to avoid soft drink. All soft drinks are improved with heaps of sugar. The more you can remove of your eating routine the better. Additionally, diet soft drink is still soft drink. It might not have as much sugar, but rather it has different synthetic compounds and parts that are bad for your body either. On the off chance that you drink a soft drink, neutralize it with a glass of water. Keep in mind, caffeine gets dried out you also. Decaffeinated soft drinks still have caffeine in little sums too and the same amount of sugar, so they are very little more advantageous either .

TIP #6: Fruit juice isn't as solid as a great many people think either. Squeeze really has a ton of sugar in it also. On the off chance that you are longing for a glass of juice, drink crisp natural product squeeze rather than juice that has fake flavors and shading. It is shockingly better in the event that you can make your own natural product juice. Simply make sure not to include excessively sugar which adds to the calories. Rather than beverage organic product juice, eat more natural product. Organic product gives your body genuinely necessary fiber and in addition nutrients .

TIP #7: Go simple on the tea and espresso. They are basically innocuous in the event that you don't include a ton of cream and sugar to them. It is the cream and sugar that winds up stuffing. Consider it along these lines, when you have some espresso or tea with cream and two solid shapes of sugar, you are basically eating a bit of chocolate cake unfailingly. Presently consider what number of bits of cake you are eating when you have a Venti Starbucks Latte – wow .

TIP #8: If you should have your tea and espresso, attempt to drink it dark. Dark tea or espresso really has medical advantages to it as long as you neutralize the caffeine in your body with a huge glass

of water. Caffeine is additionally not bravo since it influences works in your body, similar to your digestion .

Another sort of tea that you can drink uninhibitedly is green tea. Green tea has been utilized as a prescription in China for more than 4,000 years. It helps the stomach related framework and can help facilitate an excessively full stomach and it has been connected to a decrease in malignant growth hazard .

TIP #9: If you can say no to liquor, at that point that is ideal. Liquor drinks are not actually bravo, despite the fact that a glass of red wine has heart benefits, most are simply swelling. Brew is particularly swelling. Mixed drinks are stuffing relying upon what they are made of. For example, bourbon and Coke. The bourbon may not be swelling, but rather the Coke certainly is. In addition, after a couple of beverages the vast majority get the munchies and when you're feeling somewhat intoxicated and hungry you won't have the capacity to settle on levelheaded choices with respect to your eating regimen and it's normally late during the evening, just before you go out from a night of drinking, that you gorge. The general blend is simply not a decent one .

TIP #10: If you should have liquor, attempt dry wine. Dry wine is superior to your sweet wines, since sweet wines have more sugar! Dry wines have sugar, yet its vast majority has been matured away into liquor and from a load increasing point of view, dry is better .

TIP #11: Another word on espresso, that isn't really awful, however more intriguing than anything. A few people have revealed that when they drank dark espresso before working out, they lost more weight. There's no logical evidence to back this, however nutritionists trust it might be caused by the body being compelled to rely upon fat for fuel. Hello, it merits attempting in the event that you can stand dark espresso. Simply make sure to drink a lot of water amid your activity !

TIP #12: Avoid drinking over the top measures of espresso, as it desensitizes your body to the common fat consuming impacts that caffeine has. A couple of containers (if the day's extremely ease back to begin) max .

Part 2

eating great and losing the pounds

Alright, when a great many people consider getting in shape and eating, they consider eating less junk food. All things considered, lamentably, the majority of the prevailing fashion consumes less calories out there will in general reason individuals to put on weight. Why? Since they starve them to death and the individual in the long run separates and eats everything in sight since they are so darn hungry. They additionally deny them of the nourishments that they cherish. This isn't an approach to get more fit, nor is it an approach to live. You just motivation yourself push, which really makes you put on weight !

Along these lines, in eating in that spot a couple of tips that you can pursue every single day and they're not going to deny you of the sustenances that you cherish, yet treat those nourishments as extravagance things so you appreciate them significantly more .

TIP #13: Eat new products of the soil that have high water content. These are nourishments like tomatoes, watermelons, melon, kiwi, grapes – you get the thought. Those crisp and delightful delicious foods grown from the ground are beneficial for you. These things contain around 90 to 95% water, so you can eat a great deal of these and they will top you off without including the pounds .

TIP #14: Eat crisp natural product rather than prepared organic product. Anything that is prepared as more sugar. Prepared and canned natural products likewise don't have as much fiber as new organic products .

TIP #15: Increase your fiber allow as much as you can. This typically implies eating more foods grown from the ground .

TIP #16: Veggies are your companions with regards to shedding pounds. There are huge amounts of alternatives here and you may even need to attempt some you haven't had previously. The verdant green assortments are the best and you generally need to work in a plate of mixed greens when you can. Plates of mixed greens are pressed with supplements as long as you don't pour excessively dressing on and stack them with an excess of cheddar. The verdant greens likewise have a great deal of normal water .

TIP #17: Be canny about what you eat. Try not to eat just to eat. Creatures eat on nature; individuals eat when they realize their body truly needs it. Try not to be a drive eater .

TIP #18: Watch all that you expend from the sustenance itself to what you top it with. Garnishments and sauces can undermine a solid supper since they are commonly high in fat .

TIP #19: Get an idea about the sweet tooth. This doesn't mean you can't have your desserts; slmply don't eat them as a supper. Keep in mind forget that these desserts wind up adding to a zone that you don't need them to add to. Try not to deny yourself either however, in light of the fact that then you'll eat twice the same number of as you should .

TIP #20: Set supper times and stick to them. Attempt to have your dinners at explicit occasions and eat them around then. An eating example will assist you with controlling what you eat and when you eat it. Additionally, it truly is smarter to have 5 little dinners daily as opposed to only a couple of tremendous suppers. Simply eating once multi day makes your body feel as if it is starving, which packs on fat as opposed to utilizing it as fuel. Additionally, don't hold up until the point when your destitute to eat. This just influences you to indulge until the point when you're full .

TIP #21: Eat just when you are ravenous. Make certain to drink a glass of water first to decide whether you truly are eager or on the off chance that you are extremely parched. Numerous individuals tend to eat when they see nourishment. It doesn't mean they are eager; they simply need to eat it. Try not to eat anything you're offered except if you truly are ravenous. On the off chance that you believe you should eat it out of being considerate, simply snack, don't have a supper.

TIP #22: Try not to nibble between suppers, but rather on the off chance that you should have a tidbit ensure it is a solid one. On the off chance that you venture out a great deal endeavor to discover sound tidbits and not shoddy nourishment .

TIP #23: Veggies make extraordinary tidbits. They can get you through the cravings for food on the off chance that you are having them. Carrots are incredible in light of the fact that they fulfill yearning and they are stuffed with supplements .

TIP #24: Counting calories is a smart thought for those must have sustenance things. On the off chance that it is a bundled nourishment thing, it will have the calories on the bundling. Make certain to focus on serving sizes regarding calories too. An Otis Spunkmeyer biscuit is planned to be two servings, so you need to twofold the calories recorded. This is the place nourishment makers get dubious and you can't fall in their snare .

TIP #25: Work off the additional calories before the week's over. In the event that you believe you have overdone it a lot of this current week, make sure to get to the rec center or go strolling somewhat longer to work off those additional calories you have devoured .

TIP #26: Stay far from everything seared. On the off chance that it is breaded, it is better that it is prepared. Seared sustenances are submerged in fat and oil. Indeed, even after the overabundance has oil has been depleted away, there is still oil consumed into the nourishment thing itself .

TIP #27: Don't skip dinners. You ought to have, something like, three suppers every day, except ideally five little dinners. This will shield you from getting ravenous amid the day and gorging out of starvation .

TIP #28: Just like organic products, new vegetables are superior to anything those that are canned. It is shockingly better in the event that you can eat your veggies crude. When you cook them, you cook away the supplements. On the off chance that you should cook them, endeavor to bubble them to the point that there is still some freshness to them. Likewise, don't absorb them margarine. On the off chance that you can purchase natural and pesticide free veggies, that is far and away superior .

TIP #29: Don't eat more than one egg for each day. It is ideal in the event that you can diminish your egg admission to three every week .

TIP #30: Chocolates ought to be treated as extravagance things. Purchase the well done and just eat them each once in for a little while. On the off chance that you truly enjoy every piece, you'll encounter substantially more happiness in eating them and they will taste far superior .

TIP #31: Eat sustenances from the majority of the nutrition types every day. This is an extraordinary method to guarantee you are getting every one of the supplements your body needs and it avoids any eating routine insufficiencies. Additionally, don't eat similar sustenances constantly. Analysis so you don't get exhausted with same old eating regimen .

TIP #32: Try to have breakfast inside a hour of awakening. This is the most ideal approach to give your body the kick off it needs. Try not to hold up until the point that you are extremely eager. Breakfast is imperative, yet you don't have to stuff yourself. The thought is that you're breaking the quick from not easting throughout the night .

TIP #33: Your eating routine ought to incorporate all parts of the nutrition classes including starches. Truth be told, your eating regimen should be around 50-55% carbs. Carbs are an extraordinary wellspring of vitality. Those eating regimens that forbid starches are really hurting you and just influencing you to hunger for them substantially more. Your eating regimen should make you be lacking in anything .

TIP #34: Proteins should make up just 25-30% of your eating regimen. To an extreme degree an excess of accentuation is put on meat as the fundamental piece of your dinner. In reality, it ought to be viewed as all the more a side dish as opposed to the principle course .

TIP #35: Fats should make up 15-20% of your feast. This is extremely all the fat your body needs. A ton of this will be in your eating regimen as cream, sugar and so forth .

TIP #36: Eat more white meat than red meat. White meat incorporates chicken, fish and some other fowl. Red meat incorporates hamburger and pork .

TIP #37: Try to go as veggie lover as possible. This truly is a more beneficial way of life, regardless of whether you can't remove meat totally. The more products of the soil you can eat the better. The more meat you cut out, the more fat you can remove of your eating regimen also. Nonetheless, protein is critical, so be sure that your choice enables you to keep up great protein levels .

TIP #38: White bread is great, however high fiber multigrain breads are vastly improved. These breads are another approach to add more fiber to your eating routine and they likewise have a decent protein level .

TIP #39: Pork does not aid weight reduction at all. The less pork you eat, the happier you will be when endeavoring to shed pounds. Pork has a high fat substance and incorporates sustenance things, for example, bacon, ham and frankfurter .

TIP #40: Limit your sugar allow however much as could reasonably be expected. In the event that you should have sugar in your espresso and tea, attempt to locate a fake sugar that you wouldn't fret the essence of. Nonetheless, these things are not too sound either and ought to be constrained too .

TIP #41: Try touching five to six times each day. These are those little dinners we examined before. A few people shed pounds better when they never feel hungry and touching on sound nourishment things can do this for you. Furthermore, it keeps your digestion working, which will consume fat normally.

TIP #42: Don't stress over deceiving, however don't cheat for a supper. Eat desserts and your

 most loved cheat sustenance for the flavor as it were. On the off chance that you need dessert after supper, share one with the entire family. You'll get the flavor, however not the pounds .

TIP #43: Watch your fat admission. Each fat gram is 9 calories. In the event that you know your aggregate calories, you can figure the measure of fat in those things .

TIP #44: Take it simple on the salt and endeavor to slice what you use down the middle. Salt is one of the fundamental driver of stoutness .

Section 3

Shed pounds by changing how you cook

Here are a couple of tips that will assist you with losing those initial ten pounds by essentially changing how you set up your sustenance. How sustenance is cooked has the same amount of to do with how solid it is or isn't .

TIP #45: Instead of singing in oil or fat, have a go at preparing those things. Preparing does not require all the fat and oil that searing requires and your sustenance isn't absorbing those substances while it cooks .

TIP #46: Use non-stick skillet splash so you don't utilize oil. Additionally, skillet that are non-stick don't require to such an extent, if any oil .

TIP #47: Boil vegetables as opposed to cooking them. You can likewise steam them, as this is most likely the most advantageous approach to eat nourishments like cabbages, cauliflower, broccoli and carrots .

TIP #48: Be hesitant of no fat and low fat nourishment things. There are huge numbers of these nourishment things available, however they are not actually sound. A significant number of these sustenance things utilize a type of substance or starch to improve them so they taste better. Be that as it may, the body transforms these synthetic concoctions and starches into sugar in the body, which implies they are as yet getting transformed into fat .

TIP #49: Don't succumb to crash abstains from food. These are awful for you and accomplish more mischief than anything over the long haul. The transient outcomes are normally that you will shed a couple of pounds, however once you surrender them then everything returns and your weight is more awful the second time around. You can't make due on an accident diet and you in the long run get to a point where you need to surrender it .

TIP #50: Chew your sustenance no less than 8 to multiple times whether it is fluid nourishment, desserts or frozen yogurt. This adds spit to the sustenance that processes the sugar. At the point when sustenance isn't eaten appropriately and is simply gulped, you fill your stomach with nourishment that isn't prepared to be processed and it at that point does not yield the medical advantages that you require .

TIP #51: When you are cooking with oil, utilize a decent Extra Virgin Olive Oil. It is more costly than vegetable oil, yet the medical advantages are vastly improved and it merits the expense. Olive oil has been related with a decreased hazard in coronary illness and builds the versatility of the blood vessel dividers which diminishes the shot for heart assault and stroke .

Section 4

Practicing to get thinner

There are two things that you should do to get thinner and one of those we have effectively secured pretty broadly and that is to eat right and fill your body with great, clean water. The other thing you need to do is get your body moving. You don't need to buy a rec center participation to get work out. Truth be told, there are a few things you can do once a day that will kick begin your body into getting more fit and there are a few activities you can do individually to get thinner .

TIP #52: When you start working out, regardless of whether at home or in a rec center, don't be disheartened in the event that you don't get results immediately. It takes over seven days to get your body into shape and to start gaining ground. Numerous individuals wrongly believe that their practicing isn't working when it just requires a smidgen of investment .

If you push your body unnecessarily when you at first start rehearsing you can end up with wounds. Your bones, joints and ligaments are not set up for the exertion you are putting on them. Do whatever it takes not to feel that if you genuinely drive yourself hard for two or three activities that you'll lose money, disastrously the body doesn't work thusly. Enduring disapproved of people will win at last with respect to working out.

TIP #53: Check your weight when you start working out, anyway don't use it as a manual for how much weight you are losing. Your weight shifts for the span of the day. If you check your weight every day, you may simply end up getting weakened.

TIP #54: The best way to deal with realize whether you're getting fit as a fiddle is by the fit of your articles of clothing. In case you start to feel similarly as you're drifting in your articles of clothing, you understand you're eating and rehearsing is profiting you. Another way to deal with realize whether you're getting more slender is if you can begin moving where you generally fasten your belt, clearly more firmly is better.

TIP #55: When you irregularly check your weight and the assault of your articles of clothing, remunerate yourself. Get yourself some new running shoes or another join of jeans. This will keep you induced as you look for after your weight decrease goals.

TIP #56: Take a long weekend from rehearsing to offer your body a chance to rest and fix. Your body needs multi day from work once every week.

TIP #57: Three days of 30 minute exercise will help you with keeping up your weight, anyway you require something like 4 days of 30 minute exercise to begin to get increasingly fit and 5 days seven days is by a long shot prevalent.

TIP #58: Collect information on exercise and basic things you can do from your own special home. There is colossal measures of wide research open on exercise and you can pick what will help

TIP #42: Don't worry over hoodwinking, yet don't cheat for a supper. Eat sweets and your most cherished cheat sustenance for the flavor in a manner of speaking. If you require dessert after dinner, share one with the whole family. You'll get the flavor, anyway not the pounds.

TIP #43: Watch your fat affirmation. Each fat gram is 9 calories. In case you know your total calories, you can figure the proportion of fat in those things.

TIP #44: Take it basic on the salt and try to cut what you use down the center. Salt is one of the major driver of weight.

<u>Section 3</u>

Get fit as a fiddle by changing how you cook

Here are several hints that will help you with losing those underlying ten pounds by simply switching how you set up your sustenance. How sustenance is cooked has a similar measure of to do with how strong it is or isn't.

TIP #45: Instead of sautéing in oil or fat, try warming those things. Getting ready does not require all the fat and oil that singing requires and your sustenance isn't retaining those substances while it cooks.

TIP #46: Use non-stick frying pan shower so you don't use oil. Moreover, compartment that are non-stick don't require to such a degree, if any oil.

TIP #47: Boil vegetables rather than cooking them. You can in like manner steam them, as this is in all probability the most favorable way to deal with eat sustenances like cabbages, cauliflower, broccoli and carrots.

TIP #48: Be suspicious of no fat and low fat sustenance things. There are an extensive parcel of these sustenance things accessible, yet they are not really strong. An impressive parcel of these sustenance things use a kind of manufactured or sugar to enhance them so they taste better. In any case, the body changes these engineered substances and starches into sugar in the body, which suggests they are so far getting changed into fat.

TIP #49: Don't capitulate to crash keeps away from sustenance. These are terrible for you and achieve more wickedness than anything as time goes on. The transient results are ordinarily that you will shed two or three pounds, yet once you surrender them then everything returns and your weight is increasingly deplorable the second time around. You can't get by on a mishap diet and you over the long haul get to a point where you have to surrender it.

TIP #50: Chew your sustenance no under 8 to numerous occasions whether it is liquid sustenance, pastries or solidified yogurt. This adds salivation to the sustenance that forms the sugar. Right when sustenance isn't eaten properly and is just swallowed, you fill your stomach with sustenance that isn't set up to be handled and it by then does not yield the restorative points of interest that you require.

TIP #51: When you are cooking with oil, use a conventional Extra Virgin Olive Oil. It is more exorbitant than vegetable oil, anyway the restorative focal points are significantly enhanced and it justifies the cost. Olive oil has been connected with a reduced peril in coronary sickness and manufactures the adaptability of the vein dividers which diminishes the shot for heart strike and stroke.

Section 4

Rehearsing to get fit as a fiddle

There are two things that you ought to do to get fit as a fiddle and one of those we have successfully anchored pretty extensively and that is to eat right and fill your body with incredible, clean water. The other thing you have to do is get your body moving. You don't have to purchase a rec focus enlistment to get work out. Honestly, there are a couple of things you can do each day that will kick start your body into getting increasingly fit and there are a couple of exercises you can manage without any other person to shed pounds.

TIP #52: When you begin working out, paying little mind to whether at home or in a rec focus, don't be crippled if you don't get results promptly. It assumes control seven days to get your body into shape and to begin making strides. Various people heartbreakingly trust that their rehearsing isn't working when it just requires a touch of venture.

If you push your body unnecessarily when you at first start rehearsing you can end up with wounds. Your bones, joints and ligaments are not set up for the exertion you are putting on them. Do whatever it takes not to feel that in case you really impel yourself hard for several activities that you'll lose money, amazingly the body doesn't work thusly. Unflinching attitudes dependably win at last with respect to working out.

TIP #53: Check your weight when you start working out, yet don't use it as a manual for how much weight you are losing. Your weight wavers for the length of the day. In case you check your weight every day, you may simply end up getting weakened.

TIP #54: The best way to deal with realize whether you're getting fit as a fiddle is by the fit of your articles of clothing. If you start to feel as though you're skimming in your pieces of clothing, you understand you're eating and rehearsing is profiting you. Another way to deal with realize whether you're shedding pounds is if you can begin moving where you as a general rule fasten your belt, clearly more firmly is better.

TIP #55: When you discontinuously check your weight and the assault of your articles of clothing, repay yourself. Get yourself some new running shoes or another match of jeans. This will keep you prodded as you look for after your weight decrease goals.

TIP #56: Take a long weekend from rehearsing to offer your body a chance to rest and fix. Your body needs an excursion day once consistently.

TIP #57: Three days of 30 minute exercise will help you with keeping up your weight, anyway you require something like 4 days of 30 minute exercise to begin to shed pounds and 5 days seven days is incredibly better.

TIP #58: Collect information on exercise and straightforward things you can do from your very own home. There is colossal measures of expansive research open on exercise and you can pick what will help

you the most to meet your weight decrease destinations. Examine the Internet or get a couple books on prosperity and exercise from your adjacent book shop or library to take in more and how to expend off the perfect number of calories you are trying to devour each week.

TIP #59: Try to find a movement amigo. This should be someone who is as committed to rehearsing and getting fit as a fiddle as you might be. One of the advantages of finding a submitted assistant is that you have someone to keep feeling careful to them. The data that someone is paying special mind to you makes it less requesting for you to get up and run practice with them. You wouldn't want to stand up your action amigo would you?

TIP #60: When your body reveals to you it has had enough, appreciate a relief. When you have worked out for a great deal of time, you will start tolerating signs from your body. This is particularly basic when you are basically starting in your movement plan.

TIP #61: If you assemble the length of your activities, do accordingly a tiny bit at a time. The proportional is legitimate for the power of your activities.

TIP #62: Select an action plan that suits your lifestyle. Everybody has a substitute lifestyle and a substitute calling. There is no set time that you should or should not work out. If you like to practice late before you go to bed since it is loosening up to you by then do it. If you like to practice instantly in the initial segment of the day since it causes you wake up then that is mind boggling also. A couple of individuals like to practice on their supper break to take a break from the stress of their movement or in light of the fact that that is the principle time they have open.

TIP #63: Don't stay around, walk around. In case you can walk around, do it. People who are pacers are truly doing themselves a lot of good since they are continually moving. Pacing similarly empowers you think.

TIP #64: Don't sit in case you can stand. If you can stand effectively, you will devour a more noteworthy number of calories doing in that capacity than if you by one way or another figured out how to sit.

TIP #65: Don't rests if you can sit. Same thought as the two above.

TIP #66: The parlor seat and the TV are threatening to weight decrease. If you are inclined to twist up a constantly apathetic individual, don't sit on it.

Honestly, if you have to, put a not too pleasing seat before the TV so you won't contribute such a lot of vitality before it. The proportional is legitimate for the PC in the event that you're a PC fiend. A couple of individuals have a dynamically pleasant seat before their PC than they do before their TV. (This is, clearly, if you don't work from home and need to work an excessive amount of time before your PC in light of the way that your seat is indispensable by then.)

TIP #67: If you have an occupation where you sit the whole time, stand up and expand every half hour or close. By far most of the present occupations are before a PC and anticipate that you should sit. If you have work like this make it a point to move every so often.

TIP #68: Walk around while you're on the telephone. You'll get a better than average exercise if it is a long discourse.

TIP #69: Use the stairs instead of the lift or lift. These are amazing solaces, yet they make us particularly drowsy. Furthermore, it may be speedier to investigate a lift to open.

TIP #70: Quit smoking. Smoking does not add to your weight correctly, but instead it prompts unusual eating practices and fabricates caffeine dependence.

TIP #71: 10 minutes of cardio multi day is valuable for most, you can get this by unexpected methodologies in comparison to running.

TIP #72: If you can't continue running for a physical reason, by then endeavor 15 minutes of exuberant walking around remain fit as a fiddle.

TIP #73: You can walk wherever if you have time. If work or the market isn't far away, consider walking around or riding a bike. It may take you longer, anyway you're getting your activity meanwhile.

TIP #74: Hide the remote control from yourself. Remote controls are also treacherous with respect to getting increasingly fit. If you didn't have a remote, you may not turn on the TV, which infers you may find continuously powerful exercises. Get up and change the divert in case you don't have a remote or go for a walk around contradicted to sitting before the TV.

TIP #75: Do your very own getting. In case you require something from the kitchen, the TV channel changed, the mail or paper from the parking space, walk and get it yourself. Adding a touch of walking around your day will do considers for you.

TIP #76: Walk along or climb the lift with it or just take the stairs.

TIP #77: Walk around in the midst of business breaks or do fundamental exercises like crunches or curving around and reaching your toes. Effectively get your body moving more and to keep your blood siphoning.

TIP #78: Turn on some music and move. Yet again, the more you move the better you will feel and the more weight you will lose.

TIP #79: If you take open transportation, get off a square before your stop and walk whatever is left of the way. This is a not too bad technique to press in a walk when work or while in travel to another objective.

TIP #80: Do pelvic gyrations to get your midriff perfectly healthy. Clearly, you wouldn't do these with anybody around, yet they are a better than average development in getting your body orchestrated progressively authentic stomach crunches. It is moreover incredible on the back muscles and keeps you free instead of tight.

TIP #81: Suck in your stomach when you walk. Walk fittingly, yet do your best to keep that stomach tucked in. You will a little while later begin to feel those muscles settling.

TIP #82: Do breathing exercises to condition your midsection. It is shocking how breathing fittingly and with your entire stomach can truly settle your strong quality. Most by far breathe in unreasonably shallow everything considered and oxygen is helpful for the cerebrum.

TIP #83: Experiment with yoga. Yoga is a phenomenal technique to get fit as a fiddle and decline your sentiments of uneasiness. Yoga demonstrates to you proper methodologies to control your muscles and procure control of your individual muscles get-togethers.

TIP #84: Lift loads. Quality getting ready devours more fat than people give it credit. When you tackle building muscle, they begin to expend fat to fuel muscles advancement. Do realize that when you gain muscle, your scale may not be a correct mechanical assembly in choosing weight decrease since muscle checks more than fat.

TIP #85: Massage your associate. You can attempt a bit and meanwhile you will have the ability to enhance them on the heap they have lost if they have been working out with you.

TIP #86: Take the stairs two at some random minute as opposed to every one thusly. This makes you have to attempt more and constructs your heartbeat.

TIP #87: Take your pooch on a walk. Chances are that on the off chance that you're not getting enough exercise, nor is your pet. Or of course, let your doggie take you on a walk. For once in his life, let him lead you where he needs to go and as speedy as he needs to arrive. It could be a better than average exercise for the both of you.

TIP #88: Join a moving class. This could be accomplice moving where you learn moves like the tango, salsa or fox run. These moves are brisk paced and will make you move. In reality, even moderate accomplice moving is a lot of action and will condition your legs. Or on the other hand, you can take an energetic move class. What number of craftsmen do you understand that are overweight?

TIP #89: Lean against the divider with the objective that your face is close and a while later use your hands to push your body away. Do this three or on numerous occasions to broaden.

TIP #90: Swim at whatever point you can. Swimming is a remarkable strategy to get your cardio exercise and it's low to no impact on your joints, which is unimaginable for people who have osteoporosis or joint issues.

TIP #91: Try playing tennis or ball. Playing entertainments are an unbelievable technique to get into shape. It's in like manner progressively pleasant to practice with someone else in an engaged situation. You will be logically made a beeline for push yourself and you'll expend more calories, basically don't make a decent attempt.

TIP #92: Always start your activity with a warm up of around 5-10 minutes and end with a chill off of 5-10 minutes.Your body needs to achieve a specific pulse level before it will react well to whatever is left of the exercise .

TIP #93: Don't convey your remote telephone or mobile phone with you. On the off chance that it rings, go stroll for it. There are such a significant number of accommodations throughout everyday life and we generally have all that we require readily available, however this is clearly awful for the waistline .

TIP #94: If you're remaining near, extend your legs a bit by standing up on your toes and after that steadily drop to your mends. You can utilize your butt cheek muscles too, however perhaps when no one else is looking .

TIP #95: Before going to bed, strip and gaze at yourself before the mirror. Observe what regions you have to enhance and what territories are your best resources. Taking a self-stock can keep you roused in your exercise attempts. Likewise, bear in mind to supplement yourself on any new muscle tone you may have or different enhancements you've made .

TIP #96: Don't slump in your seat. Endeavor to sit up straight and erect consistently. Slumping is awful for your back and gives you an overweight figure. Make it a point to dependably sit and remain with great stance .

TIP #97: Most individuals might want to focus on their stomachs and dispose of that region all together. Shockingly, we can't spot decrease. Be that as it may, one thing you can do is a breathing activity to help fix those stomach muscles .

Take in air as solid as you can and tuck your stomach in the meantime as much as you can. Hold it for a couple of moments and afterward gradually given it a chance to out. Try not to let it out so quick that your awkward dives out. This isn't great. Endeavor to inhale like this at whatever point you consider it, around 50-60 times each day is perfect. This will assist you with losing no less than an inch inside 20 days or something like that .

IP #98: Use a diagram, for example, the one underneath to help you in your weight reduction attempts. This diagram demonstrates to you what number of calories every one of these basic activities consume, in view of 20 minutes .

*Your results will rely upon the amount you as of now weigh too. In case you're searching for a precise computation dependent on your body weight and subtleties of the activity you are performing go to iVillage.com at

From this diagram you can see that strolling is an extraordinary method to get work out. In case you're too occupied to even consider doing any of alternate activities, a great walk is a decent begin .

TIP #99: Don't debilitate yourself from practicing and eating appropriate by wearing garments that don't fit. In case you're a medium, wear a medium. Wearing the wrong sorts of garments can influence you to seem bigger than you truly are. This incorporates exercise wear too. On the off chance that you wear garments that fit now, you get the chance to go shopping later for littler garments and you can move your marginally worn bigger garments in a transfer shop or you can take them to Goodwill to be given to somebody who can utilize them .

Part 5

Beginning

Since you see how to begin, here's somewhat more data on getting more fit and keeping it off and everything starts with what you eat .

Fat and weight reduction is such an imperative angle in our life today since we are fatter now than we have ever been. "Weight misfortune programs" will grab the eye of anyone tuning in on a discussion or staring at the TV. Truth be told, that is a standout amongst the most well known watchwords looked on the Internet today .

The principle reason that we are so overweight is a result of our association with sustenance. In our general public, we will in general focus on amount. We essentially need as much as we can get rather than the best nourishment that we can get. Amount dependably prevails over quality, when it ought to be actually the opposite .

When you've chosen to get thinner, it very well may be hard to figure out where precisely you ought to begin. On the off chance that you have a solid set out to go ahead and to get thinner, it is conceivable. You simply need to make sense of how to state "no ".

Everyone is unique. You're not going to discover someone else who has indistinguishable digestion from you or who copies fat indistinguishable route from you. You may weigh precisely equivalent to an individual beside you, yet on the off chance that you both were to begin an activity and diet program you both probably won't have similar outcomes two weeks or even multi month later, regardless of whether you did everything the equivalent correct way every day. In saying this present, it's critical to understand that not every person uses sustenance similarly either. What may make one individual gain a pound may not do likewise to another. The equivalent is valid in getting thinner. In case you're a hitched lady and you and your significant other are working out together and suppose he surrenders soft drink and sheds five pounds from halting his admission of soft drink and you don't lose one pound, that demonstrates to you that you and your better half are not really going to see similar outcomes, regardless of whether you're eating and practicing in precisely the same way .

Basically the present society needs to work much harder than social orders of the past. Sixty years back ladies and men were thin in light of the fact that they needed to work. Physical work was a necessity or you wouldn't have the capacity to eat. You needed to go accumulate eggs from the hen house in the event that you need eggs, you needed to go drain the bovines for new drain and you needed to furrow the fields to develop your vegetables. In the event that you needed hamburger, well you needed to know a touch of something about filling out a calf and getting it butchered. That is how life was in those days and innovation has removed the majority of this manual work. In this way, rather we need to watch what we eat and we need to go make ourselves work out. In the event that we don't we don't have motivation to move a fraction of the time .

It is vital to comprehend that you weight reduction objectives are extremely reliant on the amount you will work at it. It is the one thing in life that you need to do physical work to accomplish in the event that you need to get results .

For the most part, individuals don't have to stress over weight reduction until their twenties, yet with the junk food way of life that we live today this isn't really the situation any longer. A large number of our kids are fat since they eat excessively cheap food and prepared sustenances. When you're shopping for food for yourself and your family read the elements of what you are eating. In the event that you can't articulate it, don't eat it. Handled sustenances cause us to have desires and yearnings cause us to put on weight. This is especially imperative to comprehend in the event that you are consistently going to be compelling at getting more fit and keeping it off .

Watching your eating regimen alone wouldn't influence you to shed pounds however. The best possible eating routine must be combined with the best possible measure of activity also. The arrangement is an activity regiment that will give your body the activity it needs to consume fat and calories proficiently. In the event that you don't move, it resembles you're in hibernation and your body just packs on the pounds, especially around your waistline .

Working out truly is beneficial for you

When you consider life in the past when your perspiration was caused by diligent work and the sun, it just makes you feel great everywhere. The sun thrashing on your shoulders and the strain on your muscles just makes you feel more grounded everywhere. There truly is nothing superior to anything working out – outside .

In any case, a great many people have moved to the city. The times of taking a shot at the ranch are a distant memory for most, notwithstanding, there are a couple of individuals who still get the chance to have that great sentiment of doing work and delivering something that was genuine and keep the pounds off while they do it. Truly, looking at the situation objectively, what number of homestead hands, cattle rustlers and farmers are fat? There aren't many. Consider their ways of life. They get up, have some espresso and breakfast, go to work, come in for lunch, go to work, come in for supper and after that go to bed sufficiently early to get up toward the beginning of the day and do it once more. Meanwhile, they get great sun and natural air and expend crisp water throughout the day. It really is a solid way of life. Sadly, the greater part of us work inside, taking a seat and still eat three dinners every day except need to do it so rapidly you don't motivate the chance to taste it .

It's an unavoidable truth that individuals in the city don't get much exercise, except if you live in a city where you walk wherever you go. This implies you need to put your brain to it and work at it. You need to fit wellness into your every day plan or you will be overweight and wiped out. That is only the manner in which it is. Exercise is the most ideal approach to control corpulence, it is the most ideal approach to control pressure, hypertension, cardio vascular malady, and other way of life related sicknesses. On the off chance that you can exercise outside, stunningly better. Your body needs as much outside air as it can get .

Consistency is vital

Consistency is the most essential part of any activity program. On the off chance that you have an objective, in the event that you reliably move in the direction of that objective, you'll have the capacity to achieve it .

Beginning is typically simple for individuals. They go shopping, get some exercise garments, get some running shoes and perhaps a rec center participation. At that point, they go and exercise pretty consistently for up to 14 days .

However, as they go, they think that its harder to keep up their everyday practice. Their lives turn out to be all the more requesting and they start to go to the exercise center less and less. As such, their rec center participation goes to waste and they simply quit going .

Numerous individuals decide to exercise in the nights, yet for some this routine is considerably harder to continue onward. In the event that you are not totally depleted when you get off from work, this is a decent time to go. However, on the off chance that you can't, you may need to figure out how to arrive in the first part of the day. It will assist you with getting woke up and you'll have the capacity to keep up your consistency .

There is a misguided judgment that activity makes you tired, however that is not really the situation. It might do this to you the initial couple of times, yet as you get fit you will discover you have more vitality. Couple practice with satisfactory rest, you shouldn't have any issue getting up toward the beginning of the day and going ahead. Furthermore, you'll be stimulated throughout the day, which will assist you with making it through your workday a lot less demanding .

Regardless of whether you don't have a rec center participation, odds are that there is a walkway outside your home and a few people may even approach a pool. Get up a half hour sooner, toss on the shoes and get to strolling, running, running or whatever your activity of decision is. On the off chance that you have a four legged companion, they'll clearly appreciate this time with you too .

15   Steps to Lose Weight

.1Think, "Way of life Change", Not "Diet "

Disregard conventional abstaining from excessive food intake. You'll just observe transitory outcomes. Make a way of life change by modifying how you consider sustenance and exercise .

.2Set Realistic Goals for Yourself

Begin with a little objective, similar to, "I need to drop 1 gasp measure by summer." When you arrive, congratulate yourself, reexamine, and go up against another objective .

.3Keep tabs on Your Development

We don't all shed pounds similarly, so you probably won't see improvement in the mirror immediately. Measure your body in explicit areas frequently and record the outcomes. This will give you a chance to follow the quantitative advancement you may not see on the scale .

.4Modify Your Environment to Be in Line With Your Goals

It'll be difficult to keep up your new, more beneficial way of life if nothing in your condition has changed. Stock your pantries with sound sustenance things just, so you need to make an extraordinary trek out for a treat. Focus on your "inconvenience times" and make changes in accordance with your daily practice, as go for an after-supper walk when you'd ordinarily set out toward treat .

.5Discover a Cheerleader

Enroll the assistance of a companion or relative in your weight reduction venture. Having a team promoter to keep you engaged and persuaded can hugy affect your prosperity .

.6Concentrate on Your Food

Stay away from thoughtless eating by taking a seat to suppers at the table. Sustenance is intended to be appreciated, so appreciate it! Take little nibbles, bite gradually, and consider the nourishment you're eating. This will keep you from the thoughtless eating that can put on additional pounds .

.7Discover Something Fun to Keep You Fit

Diet and exercise go connected at the hip with regards to keeping up a sound weight. Make practice pleasant by discovering fun approaches to remain dynamic. Go for a climb, join a games group, or take up surfing. You'll be stunned at what number of calories you can consume when you're having some good times !

.8Encircle Yourself With Fitness Oriented People

It will be a lot less demanding to remain on track when you encircle yourself with other people who share your sound viewpoint. You'll have the capacity to share battles, persuade one another, and help keep each other responsible .

.9Peruse More

Take in more about sound living by perusing wellness magazines, online wellbeing articles, and solid way of life web journals. By immersing yourself with sound material, you'll see it much

2Tbsp decreased sodium teriyaki sauce

1Tbsp light nectar mustard dressing

2tsp olive oil

4/1container cut carrots

2/1container cleaved broccoli

4/1container cut water chestnuts

4/1container cut peppers to two minutes. Include veggies, and cook for another five to seven minutes until the point when meat is carmelized. Serve over rice.

---

to two minutes. Include veggies, and cook for another five to seven minutes until the point

when hamburger is seared. Serve over rice .

These mollusks are high in fulfilling protein and can enable you to shed pounds: In a University of Washington School of Medicine consider, individuals who expanded their protein consumption from 15 percent to 30 percent of their day by day calories shed eight pounds of fat in 12 weeks .

-10Cheesy Veggie Pasta

31/24LEVI BROWN

Mushy VEGGIE PASTA

2/1glass entire wheat macaroni

1glass pulverized entire, stripped canned tomatoes

2/1glass low-fat ricotta cheddar

4/3glass cleaved spinach

1glass zucchini wedges

2tsp olive oil

Cook vegetables over medium-high warmth, at that point join with cooked macaroni and cheddar

This pizza just costs you 280 calories. A cheap food individual pie? Twofold that .

-11Baked Chicken with Mushrooms and Sweet Potato

31/10LEVI BROWN

Heated CHICKEN WITH MUSHROOMS AND SWEET POTATO

2/1skinless chicken bosom

1glass infant portobello mushrooms, cut

1Tbsp chives

1Tbsp olive oil

1medium sweet potato

In a 350°F broiler, heat chicken, finished with mushrooms, chives, and oil, for 15 minutes. Microwave sweet potato for five to seven minutes .

Sweet potatoes have a lower glycemic list than white spuds do, so they're gentler on your glucose—and possibly your waistline .

-12Shrimp Ceviche

31/11LEVI BROWN

SHRIMP CEVICHE

2/1glass slashed cucumber

3/1glass slashed jicama

3/1glass slashed mango

1Tbsp cleaved onion

4/1glass cut avocado

1tomato, cut

1glass cooked shrimp

4/1glass lemon juice

1tsp red pepper

Hurl together, and dress with lemon juice .

Avocado's monounsaturated fats may assume a job in warding off tummy fat .

-13Light Lasagna

31/12LEVI BROWN

LIGHT LASAGNA

2/1container cooked entire wheat spaghetti

4/1container part-skim ricotta

3/1container arranged tomato sauce

2/1tsp smashed red bean stew chips

1Coleman Natural Mild Italian Chicken Sausage connect, cooked

2mugs spinach

Consolidate pasta, ricotta, sauce, and bean stew drops, at that point disintegrate hotdog to finish everything. Include spinach, and let wither .

Entire wheat pastas have more fiber than their vacant calorie, white-flour partners .

-14Chicken with Cheesy Broccoli Soup

31/13LEVI BROWN

CHICKEN WITH CHEESY BROCCOLI SOUP

1container slashed broccoli

1container slashed parsnips

4/3container nonfat chicken stock

4/1container low-fat destroyed cheddar

1Tbsp cut almonds

4oz chicken bosom

1tsp lemon juice

Salt and pepper, to taste

Steam broccoli and parsnips, at that point puree with stock and cheddar; sprinkle with nuts. Heat chicken, top with lemon squeeze, and season .

Clear soups can help top you off, however pureed ones taste more extravagant, which can be all the more satisfying. (Figure out how bone soup can enable you to get more fit with Women's Health's Bone Broth Diet)

-15Cilantro Shrimp with Squash, Chard, and Wild Rice

31/14PLAMEN PETKOV

CILANTRO SHRIMP WITH SQUASH, CHARD, AND WILD RICE

8expansive shrimp

1Tbsp olive oil

2tsp crisp cilantro

2tsp crisp lime juice

1yellow squash, cut

1container Swiss chard

4/1container dry wild rice mix

Singe shrimp in olive oil over medium warmth for three to four minutes, flavoring with cilantro and lime juice. Steam squash and chard for five to seven minutes, and cook rice as per bundle headings .

With less calories per ounce than most fish, shrimp are the perfect fish in case you're endeavoring to thin down .

-16Lemon Chicken with Gazpacho

31/15LEVI BROWN

LEMON CHICKEN WITH GAZPACHO

2/1 3oz chicken bosom

1Tbsp olive oil

2/1lemon, cut

1tsp new rosemary

Gazpacho

1container stewed tomatoes

3cloves garlic, minced

2/1container onion, hacked

4/1container cucumber, hacked

4/1container green pepper, hacked

1Tbsp white wine vinegar

Coat chicken with olive oil. Cover with lemon cuts and rosemary, and prepare at 350°F for 25 to 30 minutes. Consolidate gazpacho fixings in a blender, at that point serve at room temperature with chicken .

Garlic accomplishes more than include season: It might enable lift to weight reduction and lessen muscle to fat ratio .

-17Zesty Tofu and Quinoa

31/16LEVI BROWN

Fiery TOFU AND QUINOA

1glass cooked quinoa

2oz additional firm tofu, cubed

3Tbsp diced red pepper

3Tbsp diced green pepper

1tsp cilantro

2Tbsp diced avocado

2tsp crisp lime juice

Join all fixings .

Lime juice not just adds punch to this dish—it additionally includes cell reinforcements that can wipe out pressure, battle the indications of maturing, and revive your body and brain .

-18Confetti Pesto Pasta

Confetti Pesto Pasta

 31/17KANG KIM

CONFETTI PESTO PASTA

 4/1half quart cherry tomatoes

 3/1container cooked green beans

 3/1cup diced chicken bosom

 4/1container pesto sauce

 4/1tsp each salt and pepper

 1container cooked linguine

 4/1container destroyed Parmesan

Consolidate tomatoes, cooked green beans, diced chicken bosom, pesto sauce, and salt and pepper in a bowl. Include cooked linguine. Embellishment with destroyed Parmesan .

This simple dish can be made in less than five minutes !

-19Asian Turkey Lettuce Cups

31/18LEVI BROWN

ASIAN TURKEY LETTUCE CUPS

4oz ground lean turkey

2/1container white mushrooms, cleaved

1tsp minced garlic

4/1container shelled and cooked edamame

2Boston lettuce leaves

2Tbsp cut scallion

Sauce

2/1Tbsp hoisin sauce

1tsp low-sodium soy sauce

2/1tsp rice vinegar

Asian Slaw

2/1glass destroyed red cabbage and green cabbage

4/1glass cut jicama

4/1glass ground carrot

1tsp olive oil

2/1tsp rice vinegar

In a nonstick skillet covered with cooking shower, sauté initial three elements for five minutes. Include edamame, scoop blend onto lettuce, top with scallion, and wrap up. Shower with sauce, and serve slaw as an afterthought .

Substituting mushrooms for a portion of the meat in the dish spares fat and calories. Besides, you won't remunerate by eating all the more later, a recent report detailed .

-20Pork with Roasted Vegetables

31/19LEVI BROWN

PORK WITH ROASTED VEGETABLES

3oz pork tenderloin

1glass prepared cubed butternut squash

2glasses brussels grows cooked in 1 Tbsp olive oil

2/1tsp salt

1tsp dark pepper

Cook pork tenderloin at 375°F, at that point present with vegetables.